INDIUM**EASE**   *The Silver Bullet*

INDIUM

NEW MINERAL DISCOVERY OF THE 21ST CENTURY

Second Edition

Author ~ **Joseph B. Marion**

~ Consultant George A. H. Bonadio ~
(Discoverer/Inventor/Patentee of Nutritional Indium)

Published in the United States of America

In Biodegradable Soy Ink Printed On Recycled Paper

By INFORMATION PIONEERS PUBLISHER

Woodstock, Connecticut, America

ISBN# 0-964499940, Copyright © January 2003

2nd Edition Published & Copyright © June 2005

~ All Rights Reserved ~

INDIUM, New Mineral Discovery...
~~ <u>TABLE OF CONTENTS</u> ~~

∼ FREEDOM OF INFORMATION ∼

This booklet is produced for education and research purposes only. The information presented is not intended to prescribe, diagnose, treat, mitigate or cure any particular disease. The results reported are not guaranteed for any other person anywhere. The research findings are provided to further public discussion, study, and knowledge as Freedom of Information, of facts and experiences reported which may be updated over time. There is no constitutional prohibition of health knowledge. This information has not been evaluated by any government agency. Consult a qualified wholistic physician for any medical problem you may encounter. When using new discoveries, err on the side of caution, rather than excess.

We appreciate receiving reports of your Indium experience.

*_____*_____*_____*_____*

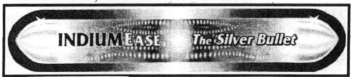

Patented Power IN Drops

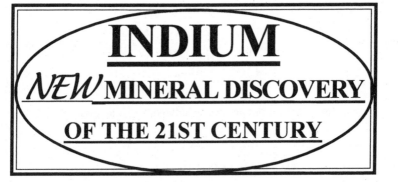

~ INTRODUCTION ~

The 7th-rarest Earth element, rare Mineral #49 on the Periodic Table of Elements, is named **INDIUM** (In) for its indigo spectral color, a soft silvery supermetal first discovered in 1863 by F. Reich and T. Richter at the Frieburg School of Mines, comprising a scarce .05 parts-per-million (ppm.) in earth's rocky crust, principally mined in zinc and tin ores worldwide. One million ounces annually of rare and valuable Indium is refined and sold like gold in troy ounces, for widespread industrial uses in bearings, transparent semi-conductors, electrodes, soft for vacuum seals and low-temperature electronic solder, lighting monitors, and Indium-sulfamate plating baths. Indium doesn't tarnish like other reflective surfaces of silver or aluminum (corrodes) - Indium gives wipe-clean non-staining surface coatings for mirrors and large telescope reflectors. Indium is the only metal that welds to glass for use in vacuum tubes, is a substitute for toxic mercury in tooth amalgams, and is used for an underarm deodorant. Indiium prevents tooth decay under 1976 U.S. Patent No. 3,937,806 of Cooley/assigned to Proctor & Gamble. Indium is used for enterochelin complexes under 1982 U.S. Patent No. 4,359,477 of Rogers/assigned to National Research Development Corporation. Indium inhibits cell-mediated disorders under 1998 U.S. Patent No. 5,763,480 of Schlesinger; and Indium's latest use is with Copper and Sulfur in a sprayed layer generating solar electricity. In short, Indium is a supermetal.

The importance of Minerals in the diet can not be underestimated. Humans are built mainly of five minerals, with "trace" amount of 60-95 others, all of which are "limiting factors" for disease-control. For instance, if one could absorb enough Chromium and

Vanadium, one might never develop diabetes; if enough Magnesium, Potassium and Calcium, defend against heart, muscle and bone ailments; if enough Selenium, enhance Immunity and anti-oxidation. Mineral absorption in humans is normally 5-20% of daily food intake, and decreases with age, intestinal and enzyme malfunctions.

Maybe that's why humans are presently thought to use only low 4 to 14% of their brain potential ... from mineral deficiencies? There must be some undiscovered, unused element in the mother Earth background that will some day become usable to unlock developing the unused 84% to 96% of the human body/ mind carriage. That miraculous mineral catalytic "silver bullet" may be Indium, a key absorbable for the first time in history in Century 21 thanks to George Bonadio.

Historically, Indium was and is not water-soluble, so is found 99% deficient in all plants and animals, including humans at the top of the food chain, unavailable from mother Nature except for 1%. Indium is not found in plant fauna or animals on autopsy over nanograms, and estimated measuring not over .005 ppm. in some plants.

That's because there are Three (3) Problems facing Indium as a nutritional supplement:

Number 1: Indium is the <u>Seventh-Rarest Element</u> on earth; there's no nuggets to be found, only scarce Indium dust.

Number 2: Indium is <u>Insoluble In Water</u>, preventing Indium absorption in food plants - thus in animals. Total human estimated daily food intake is a meager 8 micrograms (mcg.) of Indium.

Number 3: Indium <u>Binds With Any Organic Material Contacted</u>, passing through human stomach foods and intestines mostly unabsorbed, leaving 1/40th or .2 mcg. of the 8 mcg. Indium eaten daily with other foods actually absorbed.

These three facts were discovered and overcome by George A.H. Bonadio as he experimented with Indium since 1976.

Since little if any Indium was ever discovered in humans, only homeopathic "Indium Metalicum" in triturated, highly-diluted homeopathy form has been available for seventy years; prescribed for concentration, irritability, depression, afternoon sleeping, dizziness, migraines and headaches, eye pains, neck and shoulder stiffness, muscle pains, backache, hand and arm trembling, tired legs, weakness; acne, sneezing, sinuses, sore throat, fever, mouth sores, coughs; poor appetite, bloated nausea, intestinal problems and pains; urinary, and menses problems. The U.S. Pharmacopedia homeopathic Indium Benefits List parallels the beneficial properties reported with full-strength patented INDIUM mineral water supplementation; which we believe goes beyond the benefits attainable with the tiny diluted homeopathic dose, which will be further lost binding-up with any additive carrier.

Since its discovery in the 19th century, Indium as a trace mineral Nutrient supplement was neglected by biochemists and scientists, private and public, for nearly 100 years. The "Ivy League" Dartmouth Medical School's renowned scientist Dr. Henry A. Schroeder, having been instrumental in successfully removing toxic lead from American gasoline and paints in the 1970's, and perfecting spacesuit safety; luckily for mankind, turned his scientific attention to seven other little-studied elements - Scandium, Chromium VI, Gallium, Yttrium, Rhodium, Palladium, and little-known Indium - #49 in the middle of the Periodic Table of Elements. Dr. Schroeder's Dartmouth Medical School studies found six of those elements carcinogenic, and one not ... the rare and valuable mysterious Indium, legendary with White Gold as an elixer of awareness and youth.

*_____*_____*_____*_____*

Periodic Table

INDIUM is Number 49 ~ Middle of the 100-Element Periodic Table

Periodic Table of Elements Showing #49 Indium

~ Pioneer DR. HENRY A. SCHROEDER, M.D. ~
~ of Dartmouth University Medical School ~

Toxicologist Dr. Henry Alfred Schroeder, M.D. was the first scientist to design and carry out clinical studies and tests with the rare mineral Indium at the ivy league Dartmouth University Medical School in New Hampshire on batches of 200 mice compared to 200 controls, with help of assistants J.J. Balassa, Marian Mitchner, M. Kanisawa, A.P. Nason, and W.H. Vinton from 1964 to 1973. Dr. Schroeder's team eventually published thirteen (13) clinical studies on the effects of Indium supplementation in mice.

Dr. Schroeder's Dartmouth Medical School research team reported that INDIUM improved the average mineral absorption of Chromium, Copper, Manganese and Zinc in major mice glands 142%; and raised Chromium in all organs average 333% ... 90% in the spleen, 112% in the kidneys, 242% in the liver, 536% in the heart, and 694% in the kidneys.

Minerals are "limiting factors" preventing attainment of optimal metabolism and health, because their absorption is typically very low, as for Iron, Chromium, Vanadium, Selenium, etc.. Schroeder et al. found that Indium raised mice average glandular Manganese 94%, Zinc 79%, and Copper 61%, enhancing glandular performance and potential. Bonadio saw similar increased glandular absorption and functioning in humans never reported before.

In fact, it could be deduced that levels of minerals in the major human organs are proportional to, and dependant upon, the rare and hard-to-absorb trace mineral Indium, set at Number 49 in the middle of the Periodic Table of 100 Elements, a unifying revolutionary discovery that Henry Schroeder may not have realized the full impact and implications of in his toxicology studies when he passed away in 1971 after four years in a wheelchair from multiple sclerosis.

Nevertheless, Dr. Schroeder brought the human specie to the threshhold of inventor George Bonadio's discovery he coined "A Feeling of Easy Living." This unmistakable progressive development naturologic researcher Joseph Marion describes as Level-2 of glandular performance based on 61-300% increase in glandular mineral reserves, rebuilding and enhancing glands and tissues with youthened performance.

*_____*_____*_____*_____*

"Indium Tastes Terrifically Tart like blackberries or Vitamin C, And Works Wonderfully Well"

11

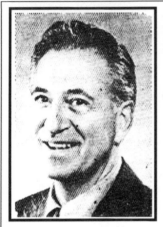
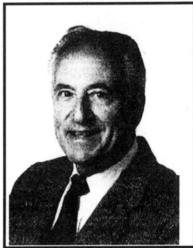
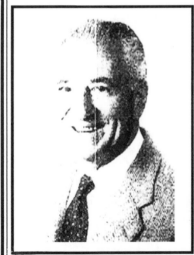
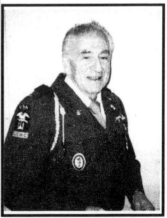

Patentholder George A. H. Bonadio PHOTOS

~ Discoverer/Inventor GEORGE A. H. BONADIO ~

Along came George Alexander Hudson Bonadio, born in upstate New York on Christmas eve in 1917, a brilliant mathematician, psychic, radio electronics wizard and inventor, having survived over twenty sure-death situations on three continents during World War II during his twenties, including playing a key unknown heroic role at headquarters for the nearly-disasterous Allied D-Day invasion of Normandy at Omaha Beach, and its aftermath, often attributing a divine hand to his continual near-miss survivals and plucky luck.

George survived bullets, bombs, mines, mistakes, malaria and his return to America postwar when two sister Victory Ships returning from World War II sadly sank with 2,000 victorious American soldiers in a fierce North Atlantic storm, while Bonadio's unballasted 3rd returning Victory ship and 1000 soldiers survived. Then a sister aircraft enroute to Seattle/Tacoma crashed into Washington's Cascade mountains with 24 more soldiers perishing, while George's 2nd plane with another 24 soldiers arrived safely.

George became a well-respected businessman in his father's footsteps, a health lecturer in upstate New York, a proficient ham radio operator who studied ancient philosphy, cosmology and hypnotism, filing several radio patents, while providing his wife and three children a natural wellness lifestyle, and established the Foundation For Health to promote natural health research and education.

In his health research efforts, George Bonadio learned in 1974 of Dr. Henry A. Schroeder's Dartmouth University Medical School studies with the rare mineral Indium on thousands of mice, and he poured over Dr. Schroeder's findings with his analytical, mathematical mind, continuing the odyssey after Dr. Schroeder's death in a wheelchair from multiple sclerosis after a renowned career in toxicology research.

George Bonadio noticed patterns, and he discovered that Dr. Schroeder's final numbers showed that Indium wasn't just "not cancer-causing" as Schroeder had assumed. Bonadio calculated that Schroeder's numbers, as yet uninterpreted, proved that the Indium had given the mice studied twenty-six percent (26%) fewer cancers, and forty-two percent (42%) fewer malignant tumors over the 500-day mice lifespan; and that the mice had lived on average about 7% longer than the controls.

Bonadio deduced that Indium wasn't only "not causative of cancer" (as Schroeder had reasoned), but

Bonadio saw in the statistic numbers that Indium actually had an as-yet unidentified anti-carcinogenic, anti-cancer function, and anti-aging factor.

Since Schroeder was unaware that Indium bound up insolubly with organic materials, he fed Indium to the study mice along with food mash, which lessened the Indium absorption. In fact, Indium's cancer-prevention effect(s) may be much higher than Schroeder reported in his poor-absorption studies, and Bonadio discovered. What does the rare INDIUM do, besides raising average Mineral absorption bodywide 61%-200%-300% and more, up to 694% ?

From Schroeder's mineral absorption figures, Bonadio theorized that Indium might also enhance large intestine absorption of Calcium, Magnesium, Iodine, Iron, Selenium, Vanadium, Cobalt, Nickel, Tin, Silicon, etc.; which translates into Indium allowing greater DNA-demanded glandular mineral uptake and function, onto what Joseph Marion visualizes as Level-2 of nutritional DNA-performance, expressing a higher anti-ailment threshhold and defense.

George Bonadio also deduced that INDIUM's enhancement of Mineral absorption might improve intestinal assimilation of foods and supplements, recycle trace minerals from the large intestine, and overall build up such body Mineral reseves that INDIUM could relieve appetite cravings, excess weight; and roll back chronic, stubborn ailments for which science and medicine had formerly erroneously thought there were no cures (concept Copyright Bonadio 1999).

George Bonadio's early pioneering work with the nutritional properties of Indium culminated with his first of three Indium patents, Patent Number 4,182,754 on January 8, 1980 entitled "Oral Ingrestion of Indium." Bonadio's second nutritional Indium Patent Number 4,591,506 on May 27, 1986 entitled "Rare Element Indium Not In Biosphere, Is Used For Numerous Healthful Purposes."

Truly, Indium manifests as a missing-link supermetal, proverbial "Silver Bullet," mid-Periodic Table at #49 unifying and catalyzing the largest two mineral groups usable in the human body, correcting multiple mineral deficiencies. Could INDIUM be safer than Selenium, more beneficial than Silver or Gold?

New York State Health Department and F.D.A. agents started surveilling and harassing Bonadio, pretending they had a search warrant under false pretense of another business inspection letter, as two agents came to interrogate and record Bonadio on his back porch. Later George was repeatedly told his telephone was secretly tapped, and his Indium source soon refused to sell supplies to George any longer. Someone had interfered in commerce. Did government agents have an interest and hand in suppressing Indium?

*_____*_____*_____*_____*

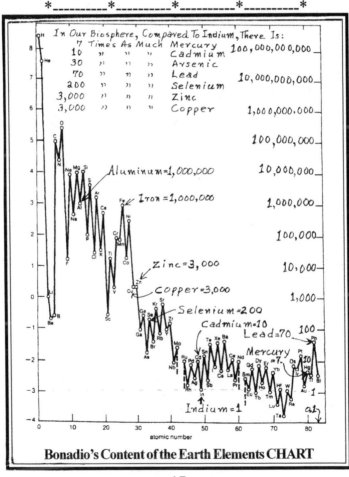

Bonadio's Content of the Earth Elements CHART

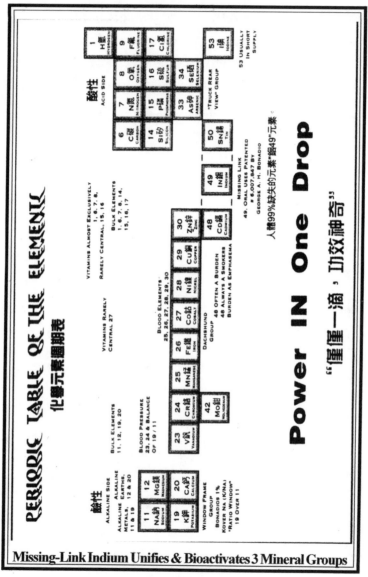

Missing-Link Indium Unifies & Bioactivates 3 Mineral Groups

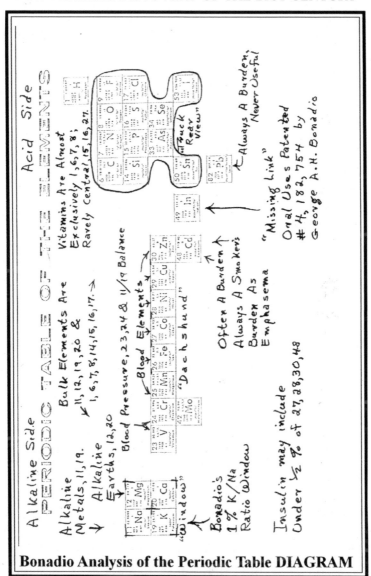

Bonadio Analysis of the Periodic Table DIAGRAM

~Bonadio's INDIUM PATENT NUMBER 6,007,847~

George Bonadio began experimenting with Indium compounds in 1976, and filed his first of three Indium patents in January 1980, another in May 1986. Bonadio's third Indium Patent Number 6,007,847 entitled "Methods For Administering Nutritional Indium" was filed on 2/10/1998, and granted on December 28, 1999 to 2016, which Patented the process by which Indium is made absorbable and usable in humans for the first time in earth's history, a phenomenal accomplishment discovery.

During 25 years of research and study, Bonadio isolated Indium-sulfate as the best non-toxic Indium compound, and the only way to absorb it was all alone away from all foods, in a carrier of pure distilled water. Having a safe track record for sales prior to 1994 without report of adverse effect, Bonadio's "Indiumease The Silver Bullet" has G.R.A.S. status, an F.D.A. designation meaning 'Generally Recognized As Safe.'

Thus, G.R.A.S. Indium is patently taken in liquid drops on back of the tongue, swallowed for optimal stomach absorption, ideally taken 7-10 hours after last eating the night before, first thing upon awakening in the morning on an empty stomach, waiting 10/20/30 minutes before brushing the teeth or taking other food or drink – depending if active/sedentary/or bedridden. We recommend starting slowly, build to normal Ind. amount in 4-6 weeks.

*　　　　*　　　　*　　　　*　　　　*

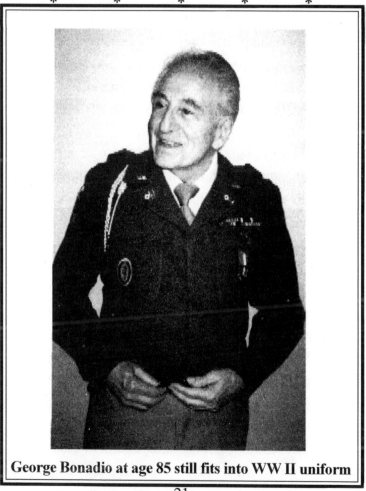

George Bonadio at age 85 still fits into WW II uniform

~~ **Bonadio Discovers Indium's** ~~
~ **GLANDULAR REBUILDING** ~

Over 1,000 human volunteers studied by George A.H. Bonadio and Dr. Schroeder's 1,300 lab animal studies over the past 40 years suggests that INDIUM normalizes the Pituitary-Hypothalamus master gland regulating 40 endocrine gland systems, balancing dozens of Hormones, Human Growth Hormone, DHEA, and many steroids. Directly or indirectly, Indium seems to restore metabolism-controlling Thyroid hormones, ridding low-thyroid (shown by 1/16th-inch pink color inside the eyelid according to Bonadio); enhancing calorie-burning to normalize body temperature, metabolism, and excess weight. Older women are prone to low-thyroid ailments, low body temperature and metabolism, Wilson's disease, arthritis, gray and falling hair, and weight gain, which patented Indium has been reported to correct.

Bonadio discovered that Indium reduced chemical addictions in 1-2 weeks. Dr. Lyons reported brain Substance-P containing Indium is as effective as drug antidepressant Prozac. Indium may lessen drug, chemical, alcohol, caffeine, and nicotine toxicity and effects by two-thirds (2/3); making drugs become processed out as toxins by the liver faster, reducing drug effects, and removing toxic drug residues from liver and fat tissues; protecting the liver, kidneys, spleen, lymph, pancreas, adrenals, et al.. Marion reasoned that an Indium-supplemented liver functioning at 2-3 times normal capacity, would process an ounce of alcohol every 20 minutes, instead of over an hour, explaining it's anti-inebrietion effects. Bonadio found one had to drink about 3 times one's alcohol limit to become physically drunk. On Indium one maintained non-drunk coordination longer enabling safe(er) driving.

Systemic glandular improvements in every main body system in five dimensions from head to toe, front to back, left to right, side to side, and over time from womb to tomb, cradle to grave, have been reported with Indium supplementation, beginning with:

1) Synthesis of Pituitary HGH for restoration of hair color, mood, thinking, and Endocrine stimulation; including;

2) Pineal Melatonin for better sleep and anti-oxidating;

3) Thyroid enhancement, against low body temperature and low metabolism, weight gain, and gray hair;

4) Enhanced Thymus and Spleen immune functions;

5) Improved Red Blood cells, Heart circulation, and reduced high blood pressure;

6) Provided Adrenal anti-stress, and energy endurance;

7) Stimulated Pancreas anti-diabetic function;

8) Liver-raising functions, cleansing toxic chemical residues, and help recovery from hepatitis-C;

9) Increased Kidney cleansing functions;

10) Improved Libido, Sexuality, and Reproductive health. May help ease childbirthing, prevent birth defects, and hormone imbalances.

11) Improved energy, mobility, endurance, and athletic performance in school children, A.D.D. youth, adults, and in Alzheimer and Parkinson patients.

12) Re-established learning and growth capacities in challenged, attention-deficit-disorder, and growth stunted children.

*_____*_____*_____*_____*

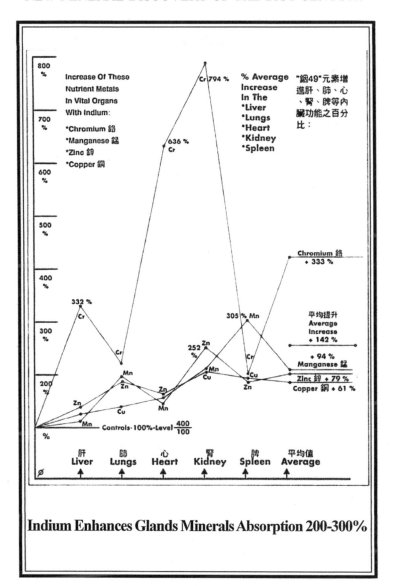

Indium Enhances Glands Minerals Absorption 200-300%

~~ **INDIUM For MOOD, WELL-BEING,** ~~
~ **BONADIO'S "FEELING OF EASY LIVING"** ~

Indium is a very deep, spiritual, powerful cosmic medicant, discovered at the advent of the 21st Century to enable essential biologic and psychological progress countering daily stresses. By rebuilding human brain master glands of Pituitary, Hypothalamus and Pineal, enabling empowerment of subordinate working Endocrine gland systems, Indium sets the stage for Level-2 of synergized glandular performance, better DNA expression capability, above the 4-14% human consciousness previously realized.

The first effects people often report within 1-3 days or 1-3 weeks is better sleep and recuperation, better attitude, vision, hearing, and mobility. Food is being better-absorbed, mineral reserves are accumulating, body fitness is being felt, the body/mind/spirit is on a subtle high performance that George Bonadio coined "A Feeling of Easy Living," enabling an improved sense of well-being (in 1 week); better mood, thinking, alertness, logic, and memory; reduced anxiety, stress, depression, and rage. This systemic Indium-inspired glandular rebuilding and hormone balancing is defined by Joseph Marion as "Level-2 of nutritional glandular performance," effects that can be felt and enjoyed mentally and physically.

The good feeling derived dispels anxiety and depression, as well-being and self-confidence improve; characterized by thinking, seeing, hearing, and moving progressively better, dependant on the better mineral reserves versus fewer ailments present.

Dr. Lyons reported Brain Substance-P that counters anxiety, stress, depression, and drug addictions, contains Indium; and Substance-P is found in the thymus gland, and travels to sites of inflammation, that may explain Indium's reported efficasy against muscle aches, arthritis, fibromyalgia, lupus, and possibly multiple sclerosis (with Chi Gong machine).

In addition, Indium is reported to reduce migraine headaches (in minutes); and give better sleep, recuperation and earlier rising (sometimes by 1-2 hours per night in 1 week).

Bonadio reports Indium supplementation reduced Alzheimer tremors (30% in 84% in 10 days); and improved Parkinson speech and motor skills (30% over controls), improving memory, stamina, and self-care longer, relieving institutional burdens.

Indium has been reported to reduce dandruff (in 6 months), improve hair growth (in 3-6 months), gradually reduce gray hair restoring 30-80% of natural hair color (in 3-6-12 months), and regrow hair in bald spots in some people. Indium also is reported to normalize tears, saliva, and earwax; and restore taste & smell functions (in 2-4 weeks).

*_____*_____*_____*_____*

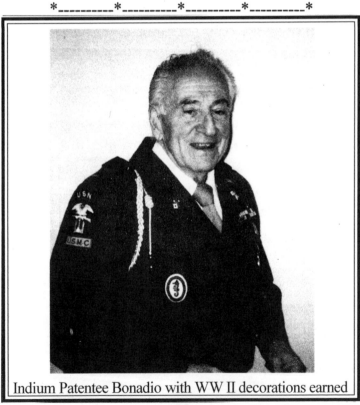

Indium Patentee Bonadio with WW II decorations earned

~ **INDIUM For EYES, AGAINST GLAUCOMA** ~

INDIUM may improve visual acuity; and may lessen glaucoma eyeball pressure (from high 20-25 numbers to norm 8/8, in 3 months) lowering risk of permanent blindness and eye pains. Careful dietary choices including other eye nutrients enhances cleansing and rebuilding processes, if avoiding foods blocking fine capillary vessels. Indium may give a slight to moderate improvement in visual clarity, fine print becomes readable again. Even shooting pains in the eyes have been reported in remission on Indium.

Dr. Robert Lyons reported Indium helped inflammatory opthalmyopathy related to Grave's disease (may be caused by cadmium), and thyroid eye disease (24%) with Indium-111 Octreotide (absorbed by the thyroid and lymphocytes behind the eye).

Element #49 Indium may displace toxic element #48 cadmium, protecting the eyes, and other delicate tissue sites.

*_____*_____*_____*_____*

~~ **INDIUM For CIRCULATION** ~~

INDIUM is reported to improve fine circulation, lessen blood viscosity, plaque and cholesterol on artery wall deposits. Varicose veins slowly regain normalcy, and associated pains reduce. Skin texture improves. Dr. Lyons reports Indium enhanced blood Hemoglobin Iron extending Red blood cell life from 90 to 120 days (33%) improving Oxygen capacity for anti-aging improvements in energy and immunity. Improved circulation supports clearer thinking, better vision and hearing, easier walking, less arthritis and immobility, stronger athletic performance, and faster recuperation.

Bonadio reported that Indium may normalize pulse in both hypertension and hypotension (leveling both anxiety and low energy); and may normalize high blood pressure (in 2 months) a half-point daily, reducing the risk of heart attack and strokes. Indium is reported to rid bleeding itching hemorrhoids (in 3-6 months).

*_____*_____*_____*_____*

~ **INDIUM For IMMUNITY** ~

INDIUM is a surface antiseptic for utensils, skin and hands (but not to be used on open cuts), and has been used as an underarm deodorant, and mouthwash.

Taken internally, Indium may enhance Immunity, speed healing of cuts and burns, may inhibit tooth bacteria, colds, sore throat (in spray or gargle), chronic bronchitis and sinusitis; counters dry rough skin and nails (in 12 months), precancerous skin blotches; and may help counter auto-immune ailments such as fibromyalgia, lupus, and multiple sclerosis (with Chi Gong vibrational medicine).

Iron-chelator Enterochelin is produced by Enterobacteria pathogens to multiply, which invading bacteria steal Iron from the host's Iron-binding proteins Transferrin and Lactoferrin, interfering with assimilation of Ferric Enterochelin, and derivative complexes of Group-3 and Transition Metal ions. Indium delays Klebsellia pneumonia bacteria multiplying time in mice, like Scandium is also bacteriostatic against Kleb. pneumonia, equal to the drug kanamycin sulfate (Antimicrobe Agents Chemother., 7/1980, Vol. 18-1, p. 63-68).

On the Chinese Spiral and Color Charts of the

Elements, Indium is classified in the yellow-green ray, positioned mid-way on the Elemental Table between Yin and Yang indicating balance, beneficial for Pancreas digestive and Spleen immune functions; and reported to improve liver function against hepatitis-C.

*_____*_____*_____*_____*

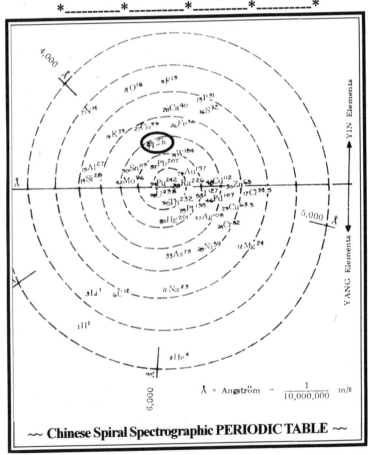

~ **Chinese Spiral Spectrographic PERIODIC TABLE** ~

~ **INDIUM For GROWTH &** ~
~ **ATHLETIC PERFORMANCE** ~

INDIUM may normalize growth rate in growth-stunted children (in 3 months), possibly by restoring normal DNA-glandular functions. Even underweight persons can restore normal hormone levels and add body weight to normal DNA-specifications, and excess weight gain is reported to be reduced.

Indium supplementation is reported to lessen Attention Deficit Disorder (ADD), enabling challenged adolescents to learn new math and language skills. Regular students become sharper, more alert, inquisitive and inspired, with less truancy, accidents, and sick days. We are looking for researchers to investigate autism, schizophrenia, palsy, multiple sclerosis, and other challenges.

Indium is known to improve athletic performance, efficiently removing muscle lactic acid wastes, and mineralizing the muscles. Dr. Lyons reported that INDIUM extended exercise performance without pain 10%; increased endurance and stamina 20%; improved running 30% further; increased bench-press weightlifting 40%; giving better energy, muscle tone, and recuperation. One Indium afficionado reports he is again matching his 10,000 meter racetimes he was running eight to ten years ago.

CAUTION: AVOID taking Indium with Creatine, which uptake raises Creatine 500% to toxic level. Allow Indium to rebuild normal glandular output of youthful days, without taking hormones from outside the body.

Indium was reported alleviating long-standing back muscle and leg pains from old motorcycle accident (in 2-3 days); and reduced symptoms of arthritis, fibromyalgia, and lupus.

Properly used, Indium may help athletes break speed and power records. A retired California racehorse was fed Indium for several weeks, then re-entered and won the next six races, while setting two new track records. The racehorse was apparantly not winded or lactic acid muscle-bound at the end of the 1-mile racetrack like the other tired horses, but cruising easily along at sprint speed, lengths ahead. What will happen when everyone takes pleasantly revolutionary Indium that might propel us into the 21st century on a higher level of conscious awareness?

*_____*_____*_____*_____*

∾ **INDIUM & SEXUALITY** ∾

INDIUM is reported to help libido and sex life in both genders (in 2 weeks), defines gender dominance, may regulate the menses cycle (in 2 months); and may lessen menopause hot flashes and night sweats.

INDIUM's improved Chromium uptake and Insulin production may counter pregnancy diabetes and premature 14% of deliveries, reducing the side-effects of eye problems, low I.Q., and extreme high or low birth weights.

By increasing Chromium absorption, Indium triggers higher Insulin manufacture, which in pregnant women converts into the hormone Relaxin for better fetus support and positioning, and full-term brain development with fewer birth defects. The hormone Relaxin improves mother's pubic elasticity for a safe, relaxed, easier low-trauma childbirth delivery (Indium could become mandatory prescription by gynecologists and pediatricians). Can we comprehend the next generation being born without the childbirth drugs, trauma, and birth defects currently experienced? endowed with Level-2 gland mineral reserves supporting improved consciousness population-wide?

*_____*_____*_____*_____*

～ **INDIUM ANTI-CANCER PROPERTIES** ～

Dr. Henry Schroeder published statistical data from his mice studies at Dartmouth University Medical School, which Bonadio reformatted and graphed showing that INDIUM reduced lifetime cancers 26% and malignant tumors 42% in 200 mice compared to 200 controls, under inadequate absorption method of mixing Indium with food. In his human studies, Bonadio reported that Indium reduced lip and lung cancer pains (in 1 week); lowered prostate cancer PSA scores about 2.5 points per day (from 313 to 85 in 3 months), and reduced reddened skin cancer blotches. Indium also rid wasting diarrhea in two terminal HIV/AIDS cases.

Dr. Robert Lyons reported Indium supplementation gave less thymus thymoma cancers, carcinogenic metastases, bone cancers; and that Indium may counter Walker-256-carcinomas, MCF-7 and HeLa cervix cancers, rectal tumors (even with non-sulfate form), neuroendocrine tumors, carcinoid and pancreatic tumors lowered 50% (with Indium octreotide). Indium reduced terminal cancer pains and lowered needed pain medications according to Dr. Lyons, but none of these astounding preliminary findings have yet been confirmed by other independent clinical trials, except one medical case where tumors became benign.

The long-term effects of Indium against cancer in humans will not be fully recordable for another 20 to 50 years, though Indium's initial reported anti-cancer effects may be quietly enjoyed.

*_____*_____*_____*_____*

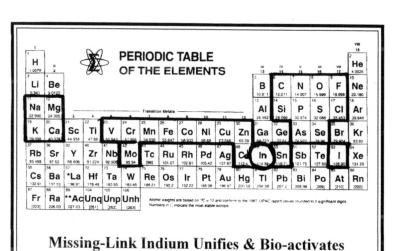

Missing-Link Indium Unifies & Bio-activates
The Three Mineral Groups Used By Humans

~ **INDIUM In WEIGHT-LOSS & MUSCLE TONE**~

Indium is a systemic gland rebuilder and hormone enhancer. Restoring thyroid and liver hormones often improves metabolism of calories, lessens deposits of fat, creates leaner muscle mass, and reduces toward normal trim weight, or allows underweight people to achieve normal size and weight. At the same time Indium's improved nutrient absorption lowers appetite and reduces the amount of food eaten. Dr. Schroeder recorded that mice fed Indium had lower body weights, especially in females, who normally put on 20% of their weight as fat, reduced to 0% added fat with Indium supplementation.

Patentee George Bonadio believes that Indium may improve male hormones that maintain trim, muscular tone, including Human Growth Hormone/ HGH; and promotes ideal DNA-determined fitness and perfect weight (even underweight persons can restore normal DNA-specified body weight).

Indium's only known contra-indication is for body-builders to abstain from using Creatine supplement, because Indium increases the recycling of Creatine to toxic level.

By raising overall body/mind/spirit energy level, Indium indirectly stimulates activity and exercise, which helps improve circulation and oxygenation, promotes calorie-burning and muscle tone, detoxification, overall physical fitness, active lifestyle, positive mental attitude and progressive outlook.

Indium users become more fit and active, able to hear, think, see and move - better and longer. Thus, elders prone to disease-borne stultifying, sedentary and bed-ridden conditions of conventional chemicalized, institutional drug & surgury dis-ease management, may delay such degrading and debilitating hospitalizations longer, later, ideally allowing some people to avoid institutionalization altogether. Indium allows ascent to Level-2 of human glandular performance and anti-aging capacity, endowing the "Feeling of Easy Living" described by Patentee Bonadio, a quantum leap forward.

*_____*_____*_____*_____*

Indium, "The Missing Link Mineral," Bio-Activates Three (3) Mineral Groups On The Periodic Table That Humans Use Daily For Natural Health, Immunity and Consciousness.
(See Chart on Page 37)

~ **INDIUM Against TYPE-2 DIABETES** ~

Nutritionists know Chromium enhances pancreatic hormone Insulin, the "Glucose Tolerance Factor" that regulates muscle-building Protein, and Carbohydrate energy and storage as fat; removing blood sugar and artery fats. Therefore, it is logical that Bonadio emphasizes Dr. Schroeder's Dartmouth clinical studies on mice that reported Indium raised Chromium on average 333% in several endocrine glands, better precursing the "Glucose Tolerance Factor" Insulin which lowers high blood sugar/ hyperglycemia; and lessens Insulin-dependance shots in type-2 adult-onset diabetes (80-100% in 1-3 weeks), requiring close blood sugar monitoring/adjusting by the Insulin-prescribing physician.

Indium may reduce uncomplicated pregnancy diabetes, which causes 14% premature deliveries and risks resulting eye problems, low Intelligence Quotient (I.Q.), and extreme high or low birth weights. Bonadio reports that Indium improves low blood sugar hypoglycemia (in 30 days), which requires artificial drug monitoring.

If the intake of other minerals were reduced to .005 ppm. (like Indium historically was because in unusable form), there would be widespread infirmity, disease, and mortality, if not human extinction. Bonadio counsels you may live without absorbable Indium, but you cannot achieve optimal longevity without this essential supermetal, which Bonadio thinks takes one to two years to feel full maximal results. The implication is that the absorption and use of many mineral elements is, and always has been, poor; relative "Limiting Factors" to optimal health, because there is no significant amount of soluble, absorbable catalyst Indium, the "Missing Link" in the biosphere of Earth. That would explain why humans are presently estimated to be suffering under the limitation of using a paltry 4% to 14% of their brain power consciousness.

Indium is not "essential for life," or humans and animals would have died out; but Indium appears to be essential for optimal disease-free longevity, and the next step up to "Level-2" of Nutritional Immunity, that wasn't available before Bonadio's Indium discovery.

Of interest is that high Cadmium intake (#48) is often toxic, but Indium (In, #49) being the next heavier element on the Periodic Table, may displace some of the toxicity of excess Cadmium.

Indium is an inexpensive and preferred primary-activator food supplement for all types of animals, wild and domesticated pets and livestock, as well as humans. Indium may empower a quantum leap in resistance immunity against ailments and diseases formerly considered or categorized as aching, nagging, chronic, inevitable, incurable, pestilent, debilitating, disabling, or fatal. The transfer is accomplished by literal glandular build-up of mineral reserves that provides foundation for better hormone supply and overall synergistic function(s).

Indium, in the violet spectrum, tested the most powerful psychic response compared to other nutritional elements.

*_____*_____*_____*_____*

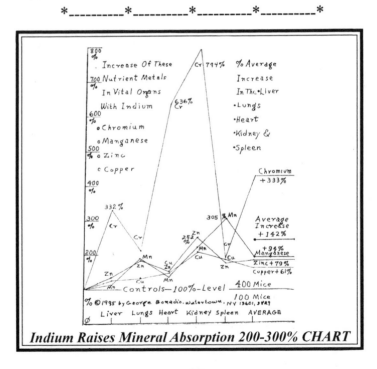

Indium Raises Mineral Absorption 200-300% CHART

∼ **INDIUM-SULFATE SAFETY** ∼

There has never been a reported case of human poisoning from industrial use of Indium, the sulfate form of which was granted Food & Drug Administration (F.D.A.) G.R.A.S. (Generally Recognized As Safe) status in the 1980's at the low dose recommended by patentee Bonadio. CAUTION: Excess Indium signs are slight forehead pressure or headache in the morning (from too fast thyroid rebuilding); or red spots on the abdomen which disappear upon reduction of daily intake.

TOXICITY: Avoid taking directly in the eyes, nose, on broken skin, or by intravenous (I.V.) injection which may damage blood;

Avoid taking with Creatine, which builds up to toxic level.

1,100 times the suggested daily amount may slightly sicken with headache, nausea, upset stomach, or diarrhea (24 Bottles taken at once).

LD-50 (Lethal Dose for 50% of mammals tested) is 11,000 to 22,000 times the suggested daily amount of 1 drop per 50 pounds of body weight (120-240 Bottles taken at once).

It is virtually impossible for a person to become Indium-toxic by consuming 24-120-240 half-ounce bottles at once.

After a 3-6 months buildup taking Indium, quit for a few days to a week, to establish body homeostasis, before continuing supplementation. Reintroduce, and adjust daily amount to your best feeling.

Indium is a conventional food element, not taken with dietary supplements, but absorbed alone apart from other elements, in the morning on an empty stomach. Bonadio estimates that it may take a year or two to experience full Indium benefits. A person may not feel the full benefits of nutritional INDIUM, if:

(1) A person is young and healthy before reaching hormone-reduction from age 30 on; Or

(2) A person has Mineral deficiencies, so there's few or insufficient elements for Indium to work with; Or

(3) A person has a weakened immune system, draining body nutrients.

Indium is a powerful mineral, do not overdo. Reduce intake amount and frequency if under severe or multiple trauma, to avoid too-speedy cleansing and rejuvenation of many glands. INDIUM compounds with food elements, so don't eat late at night. Indium "Tastes Terrifically Tart, & Works Wonderfully Well." Take Indium 1st thing in the morning at bedside, and wait ten (10) minutes before eating breakfast.

*_____*_____*_____*_____*

The Original Patented IndiumEase
The Silver Bullet, Advanced Formula

~INDIUMEASE SUGGESTED DAILY AMOUNT~

(1 Drop Contains 1.1 mg. 99.9% Pure Indium)

Place One Drop IndiumEase Per 50 Pounds of Body Weight on the back of the tongue, and swallow into an empty stomach the 1ST thing upon arising in the morning; Then

wait 10-20 minutes before eating or drinking

Suggested INDIUMEASE Daily Amount:

1 Drop for 50# (Has 1.1 mg. Indium, 240-Days Supply);
2 Drops for 100# (Has 2.2 mg. Indium, 120-Days);
3 Drops for 150# (Has 3.3 mg. Indium, 90-Days);
4 Drops for 200# (Has 4.4 mg. Indium, 60-Days Supply).

INDIUM is the Latest/Greatest Nutrient
discovered since Coenzyme Q-10, and MSM,
Experience the Power **IN** Drops.

*_____*_____*_____*_____*

~ **INDIUMEASE, THE SILVER BULLET~**

Liquid Mineral Supplement
The Original Indium-Sulfate
Packaged in

1/2 oz. Cobalt Eyedropper Glass Bottle
60-90-120 Days Supply

Available at Quality Health Stores
Nationwide

For Further Info, See: **www.indiumease.net**

**The Original Patented
99.9% Pure INDIUM
"Missing Link" Trace Mineral #49,
Is IN.,
For The First (1ST) Time In History
~ INDIUMEASE, THE SILVER BULLET~**

Enjoy the Nutrient Discovery of the 21st Century.

*_____*_____*_____*_____*

~~ **THYROID ALERT** ~~

Symptoms of too low thyroid output include feeling cooler than normal persons, morning temperature below 98 degrees F. upon arising, overweight on a meager diet, and continuously tired. Sudden supplementation of Armor Thyroid (T3 & T4, not Synthroid T4 alone) may cause a "pressure headache" upon awakening, which goes away upon walking around. Slight forehead pressure may also be experienced by taking too much Indium too fast.

If you have a sensitive constitution, take half the recommended Indium every other or third day for 2 weeks, and slowly work up to normal amount over 1-2 months. A few report up to 6 weeks of toxin cleansing reactions of tiredness, mental slowing, diarrhea, or nausea; before finding the energizing, positive benefits kick in. Some persons report benefits at 150% of the recommended amount. If hearty constitution, test Indium effects by taking 1.5 to 2 times the recommended amount per day for a week or month to see if you feel any more or new benefits; then drop back to recommended amount, and watch for any loss of benefits. Adjust intake according to how you feel.

*_____*_____*_____*_____*

UNSOLICITED INDIUM CONSUMER REPORTS Collected By George Bonadio From 1980-2000

"Indium peps up my liver."

"Sleeping better, feeling better."

"Three weeks on Indium gives less severe pain, & better sleep."

"No more catarrh, and require less sleep."

"With Parkinson's, clearer speech, more limber muscles, and steadier walking."

"Indium has given me a great deal more energy."

"I have noticed an increase in energy."

"Morning temperature raised from 97 to 98.2 degrees. Evening temperature raised from 98 to 98.6 degrees. Hands and feet feel warmer. Noticed increase in energy (restored Thyroid function). Pain in right knee and both knees disappeared."

"No side-effects after 6 weeks, at twice the recommended intake per day, at age 61."

"Increased energy and vitality - general feeling of well-being. Sleep better. I cannot see any difference between 1 and 3 drops per day."

"Better nerves."

"High blood pressure reduced from 165/110 to 126/81 (in 5 days), to 120/71 (in 60 days). Improved circulation, stiff ankle joints became flexible. On arm, regression of skin blotch from 1 inch to 1/4 inch, and regressing. Face liver spots reducing, with softer, more flexible skin. More body to hair. Clearer sinuses and easier breathing. More expansive lungs. More prominent veins. Muscles stronger with faster recovery after exertion. Not as tired condition as before. Adequate restful sleep, activated libido, and spring to my steps."

"Chapped hands cleared up. I woke up earlier. Sexual libido increased after six days. Mental ability and drive increased."

"My period is on schedule of 28 days. No more coffee craving."

"More alert, with better concentration, improved memory and thinking."

"Quickening of body sensitivity, & sense of well being."

"Less hungry, smaller appetite, and more mobile. Two hours after taking Indium, my migraine headache left. The week I take none, I observe I get more hungry and gain weight."

"General improved feeling."

INDIUMEASE, THE SILVER BULLET

"I'm not so sleepy on Indium."

"At the end of first week my appetite diminished, and my appetite more readily sated. I feel more energy, better mood and frame of mind. Lost three pounds."

"I feel better, more energy, digest better, sleep better - am very pleased with the results so far, and family members noticed the same results."

"In a CardioVascular Ailment case, recovery was accelerated."

"Lost 11 pounds on Indium. Feel more alert and awake while taking Indium."

"Indium neutralized the effects of Tylenol I am taking for pain."

"Energy levels and stamina are higher than normal or usual."

"I felt the nerves were stronger, the brain more clear and sharp, sleep became so natural that I did not want to wake up. I felt a sort of natural meditation."

"I've noticed I've been dumping a lot more poisons, detoxification. (P.S. from wife - he nearly died years ago with very severe hepatitis, jaundice, liver damage, etc)."

"My 76-year-old husband has been taking Indium for senility problems, which has helped a little, and which he missed when he went off on alternate weeks."

From a woman in 1991: "My **chronic headaches** returned every afternoon from 2 p.m. until I fell asleep. I took Indium at 1:30 p.m. for 2 days and reduced the headaches 80%."

From a man in 1996: "I took Indium for seven days, experienced **less fatigue, increased awareness** and ability to concentrate, enhanced memory, and increase in dreams.

From Dr. Andrew Bain, Effort, Pennsylvania, 1997: "I now feel that you are just scratching the surface and will find out that **Indium is much more beneficial than you ever dreamed**. My experiences using Indium are replete with almost miraculous results; (including) clear, correct and maintain **neurological hormone balance**, depression, mental disorders, low chromium, lung and breathing damage; **in learning disabled**, increasing oxygen, endurance, and sports performance. No other substance known to science can **produce these fantastic results**."

From Joy Supplee, 1997: "General **lift in energy**; the **red scaly sun-damaged spot** on my face over two years nearly gone; and returning accelerated **graying hair to original color** brown."

From Dr. H. Davis, Atlanta, Georgia 1997: "I am 47 years old and regularly play soccer with players in their 20's and 30's, and have begun to get very tired and unable to keep up. After taking 5 mg. Indium I increased my **stamina**, and can often exceed younger player's stamina, which is frustrating if they are on my side ... without the advantage of Indium. I also noticed an **increase in libido**, and long-time hard **impacted earwax** problems lessened."

From a Ph.D. in Washington D.C. 1997: "Indium is activating and harmonizing all of my glands - you should see my **beard and skin tone**, and it has enabled me to cut back on my vitamins and minerals ... cost next to nothing and I feel that I am getting a free ride on Indium. I also am able to **do much more paperwork** with much less energy drop. Thank you for making such a product available for persons such as I who live such complicated lives and can use all the help they can get."

From 43 year old food-service worker: "I needed **less sleep and could work longer** hours without fatigue, less stress. I was cheerful in the morning with fewer physical pains, bouyant during the day, and **less tired to enjoy the evenings**. From barely one, to now 3-4 games of basketball, **boundless energy**, no excess weight. I can **think faster with less confusion**. I wouldn't give Indium up for anything."

*(Reported benefits neither implied,
nor guaranteed for others anywhere)*

*_____*_____*_____*_____*

Seven Notarized Statements Bonadio prepared for the U.S. Commissioner of Patents:

From a security policeman at a local hospital: "From sluggishness and no pep I changed into a feeling of happiness inside. People now tell me that I talk more friendly and smile easier. My sex drive has improved remarkably, for my 50 years of age, to like it was when I was 25. I have less anxiety, able to sit without being anxious to get up and move, with a clearness to my mind."

From a financial trustee of a local synagogue: "I was down in the dumps at 76, but now feel radiant, more like living. I don't need as many hours of sleep, and I'm not as tired anymore when I get up; and more interested in daily affairs. Previously I did not want to get out of bed."

From a doctor, possibly with cancer: "I have a little more energy ... less rawness in right chest ... improved energy and appetite ... totally free of irritations in the right chest for the first time in several months. Off of Indium for three days, now ... discomfort again in right chest. On Indium again, no rawness in chest. Vitality much improved."

From an investment counselor: "I am sleeping about two hours less per night, and just as rested. I am more ambitious, with more drive, clearing up what I never touched before. I have such a sense of well-being that I could run back from lunch instead of walking. Mentally I am more organized, more clear. My mind is busy all the time."

From a retired electrical contractor: "Indium has cleared my thinking up. Before I had to stop and sit down to collect my thoughts. Now I can think on the move."

From a registered nurse, possibly with cancer: "The symptoms I had yesterday, in a haze and forgetful, with some numbness around mouth and tongue, have disappeared. I have more energy today, and feel better generally. I sleep very well, did not wake during the night as I usually do. I woke 1.5 hours before normal time, and felt relaxed. I lost three pounds of overweight, and still feel much better than two weeks ago (before Indium), and I'm doing more things."

From a retired clergyman: "On Indium I find an improvement in rest so that I awaken a full hour before the alarm, and I am completely rested. A very definite libido improvement."

(The above 2 sections copyright by
George A. H. Bonadio, 2000,
used with permission)

*(Reported benefits neither implied,
nor guaranteed for others anywhere)*

*_____*_____*_____*_____*

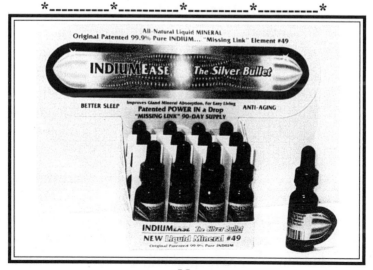

~ **INDIUM CONSUMER REPORTS In 2001-2003,** ~
~ **Collected By Joseph Marion** ~

From a husband and father: "The first 1.5 months on Indium I felt tired with dreams at night" (others feel unfocused - from toxin loosening and cleansing /drink more water & purify diet). "Then I started feeling **stronger, more alert**, good all over. My 15-year-old daughter taking Indium **gets up earlier, is less moody**, and has **fewer sugar cravings**."

From a pregnant woman (with a history of miscarriage): "I am only halfway through pregnancy, and my **premature labor contractions have disappeared**, potentially eliminating another miscarriage."

Summary of Reports of Indium supplementation in 2001-2002 were of clearer thinking, better sleep & attitude, more energy longer; cold/flu/sinus & bronchial immunity, gray replaced with natural hair color, balding regrowth, and thyroid normalization.

(Female age-65) "Last week I used the weed-wacker, and didn't need a nap afterwards ... I am sleeping better . . . not as exhausted after mowing the lawn, and worked outside longer than usual after mowing. **Indium works very gradually and gently**. Amazing stuff !!" (... reports continuing over time)

"My daughter and I power-washed and stained both sides of my 6-foot cedar fence . . . using two sprayers . . . and I didn't get tired. The prep work and clean-up was hard and grueling ... in 110-degree temperatures."

"In the past 7-8 years I have suffered **mitral valve palpitations** that would last from 2-4 hours . . . leaving me feeling tired and weak for days. When I was younger these attacks would last only 5 minutes. Well, you can imagine how happy and surprised I was when this attack lasted only 10 minutes. **Amazing, it had to be the Indium**, as I can't attribute it to anything else. I was so grateful I started praising and thanking God out loud. I got up, had another drink of water, and went back outside to finish the front of the house, watered the flowers, and hosed down the front walk and driveway with **no problems since**!!! Today I vacuumed four rooms and cleaned the bathroom. I started getting a little tired, which slowly disappeared. Most nights I sleep well, very deep and restful. I have been feeling great ! **Really wonderful and energetic**. Couldn't really put my finger on it, but I would imagine this is what people feel like when they're on a "high" on drugs. Of course it's better, for there is no coming down" (experiencing Bonadio's 'Feeling of Easy Living').

"I cooked a big dinner Saturday, made some homemade coconut ice cream earlier in the week, baked a birthday cake and had my daughter, her husband, and his 93-year-old grandmother over to celebrate her birthday. **I had energy galore**, and felt like I did when I was fixing dinner in my 40's. **Never tired all day.** What a wonderful feeling!! I don't ever want to be without Indium."

"My son-in-law has a sense of well-being and calmness on the Indium, in a much better mood, and more relaxed at work. Red-faced, he told me how much the Indium has **increased his sex drive**, and that he wants his wife to start taking it so she can keep up with him."

"About 1-2 years ago I began noticing an **ache in my lower back** kick in every morning while brushing my teeth. Just last week I noticed it was only present some mornings, and recently **it disappeared completely after a month** on Indium. This stuff is sure amazing. Hey, maybe some morning we'll wake up and **find ourselves 25 again** and all gorgeous and handsome!!!"

"I did food shopping in the morning, mowed the lawn and hosed down the patio just in the nick of time before thunder and rain came, showered, fixed dinner and never got tired until bedtime at 11 p.m. **I was amazed.** You were right when you said it delays the tiredness. **I did what I needed to do when I needed to do it.**"

*_____*_____*

(Female age-32) "I have been able to get **less sleep**, and still have a decent energy level. Also my **cycle has decreased** from 42 days to 31 days."

"I have been operating on 4-6 hours of sleep a night, with tremendously busy days and little rest. Have gone to bed after 1 a.m. the last three nights, and have to get up with my husband at 5 a.m. because the days have been so jam-packed, and very stressful. I need **the extra oomph**. Could you get another bottle of Indium to me?"

*_____*_____*

(Mother age-39 with a 12-year-old) "My daughter, her friend and friend's mother, and I went camping to New Hampshire for the weekend. If it wasn't for the Indium, I probably would not make it. The **Indium is really great for energy** and I am grateful to have it."

*_____*_____*

(Female, early 40's, overweight, had ovarian cancer, on thyroid drugs for 15 years) "Did I tell you how the Indium is working? I've been taking the Thyodine with it for the Iodine faithfully, and cutting down on my thyroid meds. After 3 weeks, I'm only on the Indium and Thyodine now. Initially

I was getting some shakes, so I did it slowly, and I was able to **wean off my thyroid meds in 11 days** and I feel terrific. **No tiredness** or anything. This stuff is fantastic. My husband also seems to have more energy."

*_____*_____*

(Doctor, female, age-65) "I think the **Indium has really perked me up**. Ever since my birthday party, when I got up at 5:20 to start cleaning house preparing for it - and was up until 10:30 with friends, I seem to be **forgetting my afternoon naps**. I can't imagine naturally having more energy just because I turned 65!! **I have tons of energy on Indium**. Now I can keep up with my young husband! Ha ha!"

*_____*_____*

(Female musician age-49) "The **Indium is giving me more energy**. I had started to get a cold and seemed to shake it off faster. All in all, I would say better on all fronts! Thanks!"

*_____*_____*

(Female librarian, age-45) "I keep forgetting to use the Indium, only intermittent use for several months. I used to get an **annoying eye tick** for as long as I can remember, which started when I least expected it, and would last for hours, sometimes days. I hated it. Ever since I've been taking the

Indium, it hasn't happened. **If Indium only did that for me, it's spectacular**. I'll keep you informed."

*_____*_____*

(Female, after using 1 bottle of Indium) "**I love IndiumEase**. Please send me a 12-pack."

*_____*_____*

"Clients report receding hair line and **balding spots regrowing hair**, white hair returning to dark color, and pineal or pituitary balanced." (J.Ripper, 5/2003)

*_____*_____*

"Since taking Indium, this is the first time I've not needed coffee in the a.m., with **better mental clarity** (after 3 days), and more energy;" and "A female in her mid-40's had terrible pains associated with varicose veins. After taking Indium, the **varicose vein pain is gone**." (A.Trumbull 5/2003)

*_____*_____*

*(Reported benefits neither implied,
nor guaranteed for others anywhere)*
*_____*_____*_____*_____*

~~ **TIMESPANS REPORTED** ~~
~ For **INDIUM BENEFITS** ~

- Effective antiseptic for body, utensils, and tool surfaces... **immediately**.
- Sore throats stopped by spraying ... **in under 1 hour**.
- Less sleep needed for full recuperation... **in 2 days.**
- Better comfort reported by ill persons ... **within 1st week.**
- Sense of well-being... **within 1st week.**
- Healing of scratches, burns & bruises speeded ... **within 1 week.**
- Elimination of pains of localized cancers ... **by the 1st week.**
- Taste sensitivity restored in seniors ... **after the 1st week.**
- Normalizing of low blood sugar ... **in 2nd week**.
- Stopping migraine headaches ... **in hours to 2 weeks.**
- Parkinson patient walks, talks, and navigates better . . . **in under 2 weeks.**
- Hard work or play endurance extended measurably . . . **in 10 days.**
- Normalizing low tears and saliva ... **in 2 weeks.**
- Senior diabetic control of sugar level ... **gradually for weeks.**

- Two cases of HIV/AIDS wasting diarrhea ended, returned to normal ... **after 2 weeks.**
- Re-establishing normal libido in both males and females ... **in 2nd week.**
- Softening of hard ear wax . . . in several weeks.
- Eyeball pains disappear ... **by 3rd week**.
- Normalization of low blood pressure . . . **after 2 months.**
- Normalizing of high eyeball pressure (in glaucoma) ... **slowly for months.**
- Retarded growth in boys nearly normalized ... **after 3 months.**
- Cleared itching, burning, bleeding hemorrhoids ... **after months.**
- Irregular female menses cycle normalizes . . . **in 2 months.**
- Re-establishing hair growth to prime age ... **in several months.**
- Ridding dandruff ... **after 6 months.**
- Normalizing of high blood pressure . . . **gradually for months.**
- Ridding dry, hard skin on elbows and knees ... **after a year.**

- Childbirth hormone Relaxin prevents premature births, and elasticizes pubic area ... **all 9 months.**
- Slower tooth tartar buildup ... **over years.**
- Return of thumbnail moons (white semi-circles) ... **in 2nd year.**
- Better distinguishing of sexual gender dominance . . . *over the long term.*
- Slower aging characteristics . . . *over years and decades.*
- Utilization of mineral content of foods increases ... *immediately.*
- Reduced lifetime mice cancers 26%, and malignant tumors 42% ... *over 500-days lifetime.*
- Male prostate PSA scores lowered consistently ... *over months.*

(The above section copyright by
George A. H. Bonadio, 2000).

*(Reported benefits neither implied,
nor guaranteed for others anywhere)*

*_____*_____*_____*_____*

~~ **NUTRITIONAL INDIUM** ~~
~ **TWENTY YEARS In The FUTURE** ~

INDIUM will be declared THE critical missing-link element "Essential For Health," and be required Supplementation against certain problems, of:

Preventing Glaucoma blindness.

Required for athletes to break world records in power, speed, and endurance events.

Used to reduce death rates from heart attacks and brain strokes.

Reducing or eliminating adult-onset type-2 diabetes' and its Insulin shots.

Used before conception through full-term births, lessening incidence of early and late births, reducing low I.Q., permanent eye damage, birth defects, and difficult deliveries.

Reducing the sleep hours for better recuperation and productivity.

Decreasing frequency of eyeglass formula changes.

The divorce rate from gender-incompatibility lowered.

Reduced need of drugs for minor ills, aches, pains, piles, etc.

The incidence of driving under the influence of alcohol will drop off, from reduced effects and increased costs.

Effects of alcohol, caffeine, nicotine, and pharmaceutical drugs will drop 2/3, with life-sparing effects for liver and body tissues.

Visible signs of aging -- wrinkles, brown skin spots, gray hair, & organ malfunctions lessen.

Retirement age of Indium-users will move up steadily for decades.

Reduced incidence of cancers and malignant tumors of all types, extending productive lifespans, and lessening sorrow of losing loved ones.

Infants will experience fewer sicknesses, & learn faster.

School children will improve school attendance, interest in curriculum, grades, memory, and sports; with fewer dropouts.

Attention-Deficit Disorder (A.D.D.) children are enabled to learn math, English skills, and socialization faster.

Growth-retarded children will develop more normally faster.

Overweight people will trim up.

Glandular malfunctions will be almost normalized.

Digestion and mineral reserves will improve.

Tears, earwax, saliva, and nail growth will stay youthful longer.

Gray hair will be partially returned to natural color and vitality, and bald spots regrow hair.

Persistent afflictions like hypoglycemia, migraines, and hemorrhoids will be reduced, as will severe debilitating ailments like Alzheimers, Parkinsons, multiple sclerosis, hepatitis, glaucoma, diabetes, immune compromises, and thyroid problems, etc. Elderly bound to wheelchairs, homes, hospitals, and institutionalizations will drop off.

Overall, productivity of Indium-users will rise dramatically, with fewer sick days, accidents, insurance costs, premature deaths; and better comprehension, mobility, ease-of-living, and spirituality; using more original glandular power supplied by Mother Nature.

(Reported benefits neither implied, nor guaranteed for others anywhere)

*_____*_____*_____*_____*

~~ Chronological **BIBLIOGRAPHY** ~~

Dr. Henry Schroeder, Scandium, Chromium ... Indium in Mice, Effects on Growth & Lifespan, Journal of Nutrition, Oct. 1971, 101(10), 1431-1438.

Dr. Henry A. Schroeder, Journal of Nutrition, 104, 157-168.

Dr. Henry A. Schroeder & A.P. Nason, Interactions of Trace Metals in Mouse Tissues, Journal of Nutrition, Feb. 1976, 106(2), 198-203.

Eric Underwood, Trace Elements in Human & Animal Nutrition, 4th Ed., Academic Press, N.Y., 1977.

Walter Mertz, Trace Elements in Human & Animal Nutrition, 5th Ed., Academic Press, N.Y., 1986.

George A. H. Bonadio, Oral Ingestion of Indium, January 8, 1980, U.S. Patent Number 4,182,754.

George A. Bonadio, Rare Element Indium Not In Biosphere, Used for Numerous Healthful Purposes, May 27, 1986, U.S. Patent Number 4,591,506.

George A. Bonadio, Methods For Administering Nutritional Indium, U.S. Patent Number 6,007,847, Dec. 28, 1999.

George A. H. Bonadio The Missing Link Nutritional Trace Element Has Been Found ... Impressive, 2000.

George A. H. Bonadio How Would It Be If We Found A New Nutritional Trace Element?, 2000.

Joseph B. Marion, <u>Anti-Aging Manual</u>, 3rd Ed., 1,742 pgs. Information Pioneers Publisher, (1999)-2003, pgs. 151-152.

Dr. Robert Lyons, <u>Indium, The Missing Link Mineral</u>, New Health Press, 2001; and, <u>The Anti-Aging Health-Promoting Miracle Indium</u>, 2004, Banner Health Bks.

*_____*_____*_____*_____*

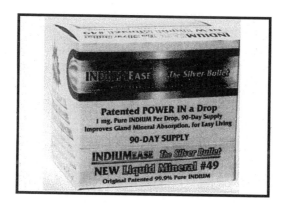

~INFRINGERS PIRATING BONADIO'S PATENT~

A ground-breaking nutritional Patent brings out the best, and the worst, in various people. Upon Bonadio receiving his December 28, 1999 Indium Patent, he was approached by whom we have found to be unscrupulous individuals: (1) **Gordon Glenn Melcher and Leslie Nachman of East Park Research Inc.** and **EPR LLC** based in Las Vegas, Nevada, who market an Olive extract 'Lenolate' product line after its development controversy and pullout by several doctors.

Gordon Melcher has a history of fraud, and was convicted of violating Title 18 U.S. Code Section 1014 by making false statements in the performance of racketeering crimes of accepting $450,000 kickbacks for million dollar loans in 1983 when he worked for Irving Savings Bank in Dallas, Texas jurisdiction (contributing to its bankruptcy), for which he plead guilty and was convicted 12/14/1988 in Dallas District Court Case No. CR3-88-153-G, fined $6,000, with $1.6 million due in restitution, 2,000 hours of community service, and five years probation.

While an insolvent, bankrupt, evasive felon over a decade, Melcher plagiarized Dr. Morton Walker's Olive Leaf book, for which Dr. Walker sued Melcher/Nachman et al. for copyright infringement. After heavy legal expenses by each side, the parties came to a mutual cease-litigation agreement, whereby Melcher coerced Dr. Walker to a non-disclosure agreement of any Indium material Melcher showed Dr. Walker (which copyrighted material Melcher had pilfered from Bonadio). Renowned Dr. Walker was thus gagged never to write or talk about the benefits of Indium for the rest of his life, unless Melcher owns the intellectual property, a gag-agreement against Amendment 1st freedom of speech in restraint of trade for monopoly.

February to July 2000, while still insolvent and bankrupt from the bank fraud case, Melcher/Nachman under the disguise of East Park Research Inc. began negotiations with George Bonadio to purchase an exclusive worldwide license to manufacture and sell Bonadio's patented Indium products. After removing many fair provisions of the proposed contract, including removing the up-front payment of any valuable consideration, tricking New York-based 83-year old Bonadio into litigation venue in Nevada, and enslaving Bonadio into giving all his future Indium research, inventions and new patents to them for free for life.

Over 12 years Melcher paid a petty $2,650 - peanuts out of 1.6 million restitution due, then made a settlement offer to the F.D.I.C. receiver in the bank fraud case, arranging to pay a mere $25,000 in cash on 6/15/2000 in lieu of the 12-year pending $1.6 million restitution due. At the last minute in the final proposed Indium contract with the elder Bonadio, Melcher and Nachman set up a front company and pulled a switcheroo inserting look-a-like "EPR LLC" to hold the worldwide license on 7/17/2000. This intentional fraud was to allow EPR LLC to secretly sell its manufactured Indium-XL products to its sister company East Park Research Inc. for lowest cost price of $5 per bottle instead of wholesale or retail sales, thus defrauding

Bonadio out of 10% royalty due on associate Dr. Lyons' 8,000 undisclosed East Park European sales at $300 per bottle (cheating Bonadio 60 to 1), and defrauding Bonadio on East Park undisclosed American sales since 2001 at $89 per bottle (cheating Bonadio 18 to 1 on royalties).

Even the first three $3,000 monthly advance royalties were not paid on time, until Bonadio terminated the contract December 4, 2000. Infringer Melcher/EPR continued manufacturing and selling patented Indium products, and then sued Bonadio for infringing on their terminated contract 2.5 years later, hauling the 85-year old patentee into federal court lawsuit in Nevada, illegally serving the lawsuit paperwork on Bonadio by Fed Ex delivery, and deleting the New York litigation Venue-clause page from the lawsuit Exhibit papers, as well as ignoring/secreting seven Termination Notices. Felon Melcher and associate Nachman, besides trying to steal the Indium Patent, are threatening to steal Bonadio's home and assets, using their pirated and undeclared Indium revenues to beat Bonadio into submission. EPR has yet to give patentor Bonadio any of six true and accurate semi-annual financial accountings after over three years of secret sales in fraudulent violation of the contract. By May 2003 forced by court discovery, Melcher/EPR admitted to just over a half-million dollars in Indium sales, indicating ten million dollars retail, and serious royalty cheating.

The Melcher/EPR/East Park Research's infringing Indium-XL product is a one-drop overdose suitable only for a 200-pound person, it is too strong for lesser weight people, whom it may injure. Buyers Beware! Other EPR agents selling pirated over-dose Indium-XL at extortionate $89 or less per tiny 1/8 oz. bottle, include:

(2) **Dr. Robert Lyons**, of Budapest, Hungary:

(3) **Ron Pellegrini, Vital-Nutrients**, Chicago, Illinois:

(4) **Harry Bartz & Rob Spinnler, Life Giving Products**.

We strongly recommend prospective Indium users beware and boycott the Melcher/Nachman/EPR/East Park Research infringing, elderly-abusing, racketeering enterprise.

BEWARE OF COPYCAT PIRATED IMITATIONS

Indium water products that are neither patented, nor Generally Recognized As Safe products of G.R.A.S. status; made with undisclosed Indium compounds subjected to unknown molecular mutations, have unverified questionable nutrient properties. Some allegedly are lasered for possible toxicity in a non-GRAS form; others in tasteless "homeopathic," "monatomic," or "energetic" dose packaged in xeno-estrogen leachable toxic plastic containers, or taken by ineffective atomizer.

Most Indium copycats parrot the benefits of Indium-sulfate, illegally using Bonadio and Indiumease copyrighted website information for profit with neither permission nor proven association with substantiated claims. Buyers beware! Use caution with non-GRAS, unproven products with no credible reputation, no clinical studies, no testimonial reports, no track record, of possible disappointing toxic effect. Such untested products may give safe Indium-sulfate vendors a bad name if a copycat product injures someone. We strongly recommend prospective Indium users Exercise Caution With Copycat Indium Products of dubious health effect, claiming patented benefits. Chose the Patented Bonadio Indiumease.

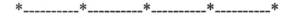

The Indium molecule is 2-3 Angstroms wide, comprised of 49 Protons surrounded by five Orbits of 66 Electrons. Lasering or altering the fundamental Natural Indium Molecule gives an unknown, unnatural, unpredictable, possibly hazardous, fractured molecule that may have detrimental effects or cause free radical damage. See the Indium Molecular Specifications on pages 76-77. Beware of non-patented, non-GRAS altered Indium products that could be hazardous to your health.

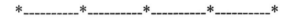

CAUTION: Non-GRAS, non-sulfate, non-patented copycat indium products may be hazardous to your health! and are not to be confused with safe Indiumease. Report any questionable, untested products to our Indium Hot-Line Telephone No. 310-589-5278 for investigation. If you report and send us info of an unknown imitation indium product, earn a free bottle reward of the Original Patented INDIUMEASE THE Silver Bullet.

~ NOTES ~

INDIUM MOLECULAR SPECIFICATIONS & ATOMIC STRUCTURE

Atomic Radius: 2 Angstroms
Atomic Volume: 15.7 cm^3/mol
Covalent Radius: 1.44 Angstroms
Cross Section: 194 barns
Electron Configuration: $1s^2\ 2s^2p^6$ c $3s^2p^6d^{10}\ 4s^2p^6d^{10}\ 5s^2p^1$

SHELL MODEL

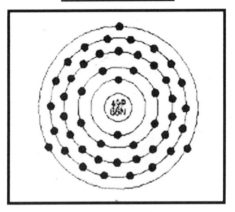

Ionic Radius: 0.8 Angstrom
Filling Orbital: $5p^1$
Number of Electrons: 66 (most common, stable nuclide)
Number of Protons: 49
Oxidation States: 3

*_____*_____*_____*_____*

INDIUM'S CHEMICAL PROPERTIES

Electrochemical Equivalent: 1.428 g/amp-hr.
Electron Work Function: 4.12 eV
Electronegativity: 1.78 (Pauling)
Heat of Fusion: 3.263 k/mol
Incompatibles: Dinitrogen tetraoxide + acetonitrile,
               Mercury II, bromide at 662 deg. F.
               Sulfur mixtures ignite when heated
Ionization Potential: First: 5.786
               Second: 18.869
               Third: 28.03
Valance Electron Potential: 54 -eV

INDIUM'S PHYSICAL PROPERTIES

Atomic Mass Average: 114.82
Boiling Point: 2,346^K., 2,073^C., 3,763^F.
Coefficient of Lineal Thermal Expansion: 0.0000248 cm/^C.
Conductivity: Electrical: 0.116 10^6/cm
             Thermal: .816 W/cm^K.
Density: 7.31 g/cc @ 300^K.

*_____*_____*_____*_____*

SEE

THE <u>ONLY NUTRITIONAL REFERENCE</u>

<u>IN THE WORLD</u> AS OF 2003

WITH RESEARCH INFORMING

THE PUBLIC ABOUT INDIUM

<u>ANTI-AGING MANUAL</u>

<u>The Encyclopedia of Natural Health</u>
3rd Revised Edition 2003, 1,742 Pgs.

By Joseph B. Marion

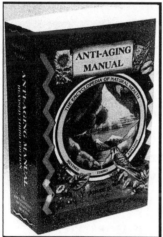

ANTI-AGING MANUAL
Unsolicited TESTIMONIALS

"After looking over a copy, all I can say is <u>excellent</u>, very accurate." J.Foran, Tolland, Ct., 4/99.

"The content of the book is excellent and will be of great use in my clinical practice." Dr. J. Power, Croydon, Victoria, Australia, 5/29/99.

"I have been researching for over 35 years and I must say, your <u>Anti-Aging Manual</u> is the best. NO ONE and I repeat - NO ONE has accomplished so great a task as yours! The Manual is so detailed and comprehensive that sometimes I find myself saying, 'Certainly Marion hasn't covered this element - but sure enough, there it is! You are to be congratulated for such an astounding Manual. I have and shall continue to recommend your Manual to others." Dr. H. Davis, Los Angeles, California, 6/99.

"I am delighted even more about the book. I have 300+ books and I know if I ever have to downsize, Joseph's book will be the 1st one saved." Linda, Boulder, Colorado, 8/99.

"Fantastic Manual, could only have been done with a huge computer memory." G. Ring, Pa., 8/13/99.

"Please tell Mr. Marion I love his book. I thank him

for writing such an all-inclusive tome on health."
L. Hotten, San Diego, California, 12/20/99.

"Your wonderful book." C. Hoeft, Houston, Texas, 12/17/99.

"Let me congratulate Joseph Marion for writing such a thorough and comprehensive resource - The Anti-Aging Manual. I am so excited and impressed with your book. Let me commend you on producing such a wonderful resource." A. Tate, Heathridge, Western Australia, 5/18/2000.

"I want you to know that I have gained much from your Anti-Aging Manual, and thusly many others as well because of you. Thank you muchly!!!" V. Maxwell, Park City, Utah, 6/25/2000.

"I am reading the Anti-Aging Manual day by day. What an extraordinary accomplishment for one man to do." R. Redeen, Pennsylvania, 12/6/2000.

"Several months ago I visited the Sunrise Trading Company, who shared your amazing book the Anti-Aging Manual with me." S. Belland, Milford, Massachusetts, 2/5/2001.

"We have used your book as our 'bible' of information. We have found it to be truthful and to the point. Thank you for all your hard work. We would like to use some of the information stated in your book in our explanations of what is in our products" (referring to HGH). D. Donovan, D.D.C., San Clemente, Cal, 8/21/01.

"I always appreciate the great book you have, the Anti-Aging Manual, Joe. It's really the best I've ever seen in this industry. I use it all the time, and recommend it to our customers." J. Pollard, Edge of the Woods Natural Foods Market, New Haven, Connecticut, 9/15/2001.

"Thanks for all of your work in publishing such an incredible book." D. Perschon, Salt Lake City, Utah, 1/22/02.

"I use your Anti-Aging Manual as a reference guide all of the time. I'm a natural health care and environmental stress consultant. People don't yet realize the trauma that occurred to our Health by the (911). On Cape Cod we all became very ill, and are lucky to have survived this event. The technological Stress and Electromagnetic Pollution sections (in Anti-Aging Manual) were a guide for me to identify the worst offenders to our health on Cape Cod, battleground of military radar, satellites, microwaves, cell phones, et al." Doctor, Monument Beach, Mass., 5/20/02.

"This book is the definitive guide about natural medicine. Very comprehensive, yet, for the most part, extremely easy to understand. This is a must for individuals with cancer and immune disorders, as well as anyone wanting to stave off the effects of environmental health hazards." Stdenzyme@aol.com, Bremen, Georgia.

"The scope of this book is amazing! The entire content and layout is easy to use, the amount of information contained within is amazing. It is without doubt the most comprehensive of its kind. I recommend this book to anyone who wants a more complete understanding of herbs, vitamins, diet, etc. I have had the pleasure of meeting and discussing this book with the author, Joseph B. Marion, who is very knowledgeable in this field, and should be commended on his hard work in putting this manual together. It's long overdue in coming." J. Barlow, New Hampshire.

--------------------*----------*----------*

The World's Number 1 Natural Health Reference ~ Anti-Aging Manual ~ was the only book in the world up to the year 2001 and beyond to write up the nutritional properties of Indium supplementation; showing The Encyclopedia of Natural Health seriously beyond any nutritional reference available upon entering the 21st Century.

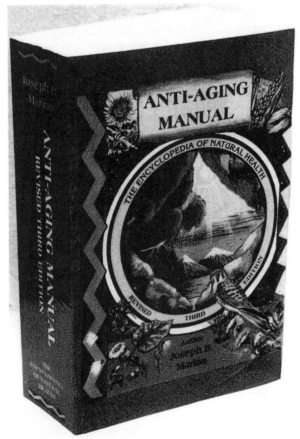

Everybody deserves an Anti-Aging Manual 2003.
Knowledge Is Your Best Insurance,
Operate Under Laws of Consciousness, not accident.

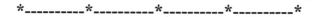

SEE Websites

www.indiumease.net

&

www.antiage.com

*_____*_____*

**The information presented in this work is not intended to
prescribe, diagnose, treat, mitigate, or cure any particular
disease. The results reported are freedom of information,
sovereignty, and science that are not guaranteed for any
other person anywhere. Consult a qualified physician for
any medical problem you may encounter.**

*_____*_____*_____*_____*

INDIUMEASE, THE SILVER BULLET

- NOTES -